..."If you want different results don't continuous doing the same..."

Albert Einsten

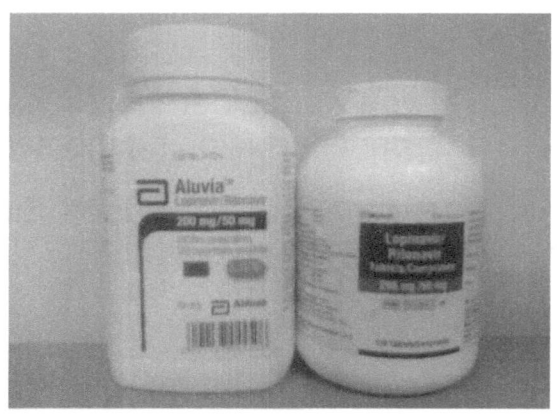

THE POLYPHARMACY IN THE TREATMENT WITH ANTIRETROVIRAL MEDICATION

JUAN E. CALDERIN CAMPBELL

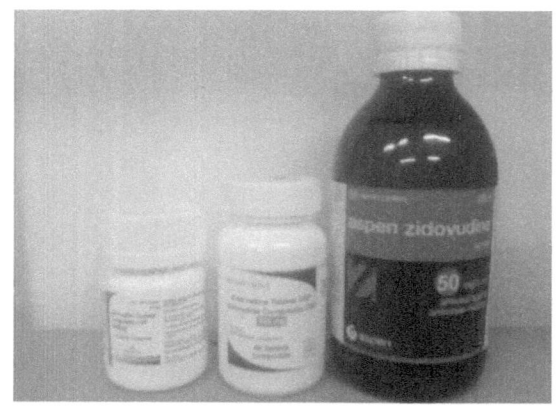

JUAN E. CALDERIN CAMPBELL

Bachelor degree in Pharmaceutical Services

RUNDU INTERMEDIATE STATE HOSPITAL.

Pharmacist of the Center for Disease Control 2017

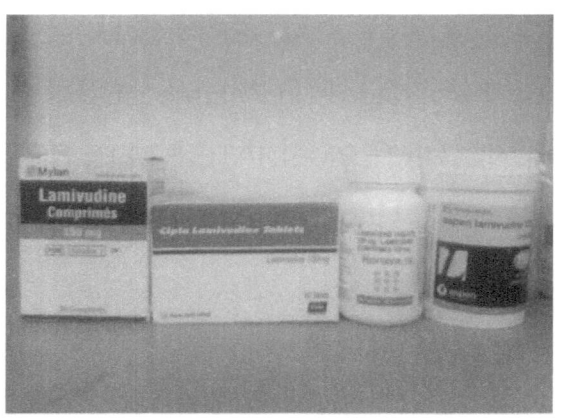

I want to dedicate this book to the commander in chief Fidel Castro Ruz and to the president Samuel Daniel Shafiishuna Sam Nujoma for to made possible the existence of this health system.

To the ladies Belkis Campbell Walter and Emma Walter Gaile for all the love that they gave me and for to teach me the English language.

To Simon Nduuviteko Carvalho and Soke Munyenga Andreas my first colleagues in Namibia.

To all my patients from Afrika for to increase my human sensibility.

To Rosalia Nargunthi (Ndeshi) my first friend in Namibia.

To the coronel Keneth Muatara for to put his life in the service of Namibia.

To all the people who are living with HIV/AIDS all over the world and to our lord Jesus Christ who will help all of us to save more lives.

To all of you

Thank you

Content

Introduction / 13

Some necessary concepts / 21

What is HIV? / 21

What is AIDS? / 21

What is an antiretroviral drug ? / 22.

Entry inhibitors / 22

Nucleoside reverse transcriptase inhibitors (NRTI) / 23

Nucleoside reverse transcriptase inhibitors (NRTI) / 23

Non-Nucleoside reverse transcriptase inhibitors (NNRTI) / 23

Integrase inhibitors / 23

Protease inhibitors / 24

What is HAART? / 24

What is therapy ? / 24

What are the lines of treatment? / 24

What is the adherence ? / 25

What are the side effects? / 25

What is the adverse drug reaction? / 25

What is the viraload? / 25

What is de CD4? / 26

What is the treatment failure? / 26

Fixed-dose combinations / 26

What is PEP, Postexposure prophylaxis)? / 27

General rules for the conservation of a medication / 29

Rules of gold to take a correct adherence to the medication / 30

Basic orientations to the patient for the correct use of the antiretroviral drugs / 32

Some antiretroviral drugs its abbreviations and side effects / 34

What is a antiretroviral drug ?. / 36

Nucleoside/Nucleotide Reverse Transcriptase Inhibitors (NRTIs) / 37

Some examples of this group of the antiretroviral medicines are / 37:

Non-nucleoside Reverse Transcriptase Inhibitors (NNRTIs / 37

Protease Inhibitors / 37

Fixed-Dose Combinations / 39

Some antiretroviral medicines and its side effects / 41

chapter two. Polypharmacy (a simple explanation about the treatment with ARV) / 59

Wihch are the causes of the polypharmacy / 59

Polypharmacy and the RDP (related drugs problems) / 61

Well practice of the prescription for to avoid the polypharmacy / 62

Antiretroviral therapy for adults patients who are in PEP / 64

Antiretroviral Therapy for Adults

patients who are living with HIV and not tolerate the EFAVERENZ.

Technically in FIRST LINE / 69

Discussion / 76

Some controversial Situations/ 77

Conclusions / 78

Recommendations / 79

Chapter three. self-medication and the toxicity of the paracetamol / 80

Toxicity of the paracetamol / 51

Toxicity / 59

The use and the abuse of the paracetamol in patients who are living with HIV / 62

The self medication problems / 85

Situation at the pharmacy / 86

Why paracetamol should be take only

under medical prescription / 87

Orientations for the correct use of the paracetamol / 89

A revision of the side effects of the antiretroviral therapy / 91

Some factors that can predispose individuals to adverse effects or side effects of the ARV medications / 92

Abbreviations / 93

Descriptions of some adverse drugs reactions of the antiretroviral drugs / 97

A grafic testimony about HIV and its Consequences / 100

About the author / 112

References / 117

INTRODUCTION

The polypharmacy has been defined as the use of multiple medications for the treatment of a patient's medical conditions. This criteria suggests that the patient is using more medication than the quantity of the medications that has been indicated by the physician and also that the number of medicines taken by a patient that can constitutes polypharmacy has not been defined.

The treatment with antiretroviral therapy is based in a brand of 3 of 4 medicines in a combination where each one of them are having a purpose and where the goal of the treatment is impossible without this combination, and for that reason based in one of the concepts of polypharmacy, we can understand this treatment as a practice of polypharmacy itself.

The medication of the patient who are living with HIV/AIDS is having two branches.

Number one: The basic treatment with the antiretroviral drugs (ARVs).

Number two: The complementary treatment (Medicines for to avoid the opportunists diseases and for to treat another conditions of the patients).

The polypharmacy has been a very controversial situation when the physician treats a disease because the doctor is obligated to use several drugs for to treat the patient and to reverse its condition to the health again.

Sometimes is very difficult to understand the quantity of drugs that a patient can take at the same time and the high risk of side effects and interactions between the medicines that can affect this person.

In this small book, i want to show this risk and also the risk of the apparition of the secondary disease that can appear in these patients as a consequence of the polypharmacy.

For example most of the persons who are taking a lot of drugs can experience the side effects of each drug and the interactions between these drugs and another consequences as the gastritis and the peptic ulcer for to drink several medicines for example with the stomach empty which use to occur very often in the poor persons.

We can say that this situation can be a serious problem taking into account that the patients must take this drugs for the rest of their life until the patients die or until a definitive vaccine appear for to cure this disease.

This book has been structured in topics like: Some necessary concepts in order to initiate the reader in this new world, some antiretroviral drugs for to show some of the antiretroviral medicine that we use in our daily work, the polypharmaccy in the treatment with the antiretroviral medication, and the toxicity of the paracetamol which shows how important is to know the clinical condition and description of the side effects of the antiretroviral drugs. At the same time we shows a graphic testimony of some common diseases in our patients.

The polypharmacy in the patients who are living with HIV/AIDS is something that we can't avoid because the treatment for this disease requires always more that 3 or 5 different drugs and the patients always have a complementary treatment; in other hand this patients use to practice the self-medication specially with pain killer like the paracetamol (Panado) or the ibuprofen (Brufen).

Once again I have to say that this criteria is very controversial because some professionals assumes that there is nor polypharmacy just because these medicines appears in a fix dose combination; in this case

I have to explain that in one tablet like for example in the Atripla, the patient is taking just one tablet but is taking at the same time three different medicines. That is to say, that the patient can keep a better adherence to the medication because is taking just one tablet but the liver is processing three different metabolites which increase at the same time the quantity of the side effects, and in this case our concern is this one and not just the quantity of tablets. That's why, polypharmacy is really a very controversial topic in the patients who are taking antiretroviral drugs.

Although the previous presentation i think that the physicians and all the staff must understand this topic not as a normal situation and they must understand it as a branch of our science where is necessary to make researches for to study and to learn in order to increase our experience and our knowledge and to increase with this one the quality of life these human been.

Sincerely I think that the polypharmacy is a very important topic and a very closely phenomenon into the patient's life and for that reason we must put our time in the service of the investigation about it.

Is necessary to say that all the pictures that I present in this book has been taken from internet collection and from some presentations of the Ministry of health and social services of Namibia using the formal and allowed linkes.

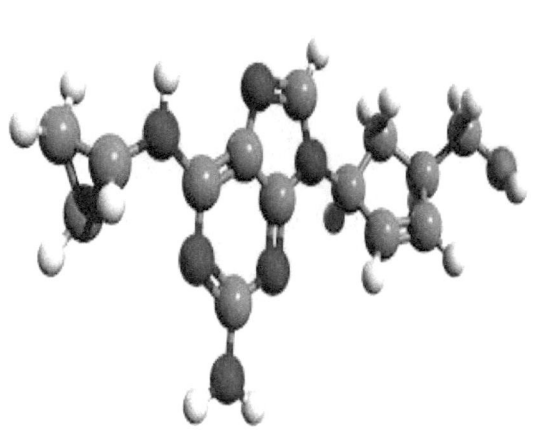

CHAPTER ONE
SOME NECESSARY CONCEPTS

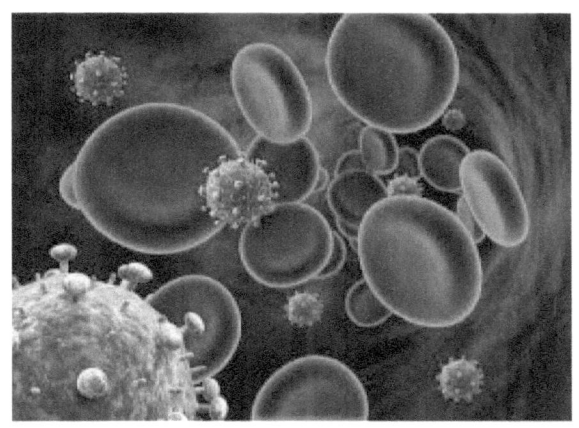

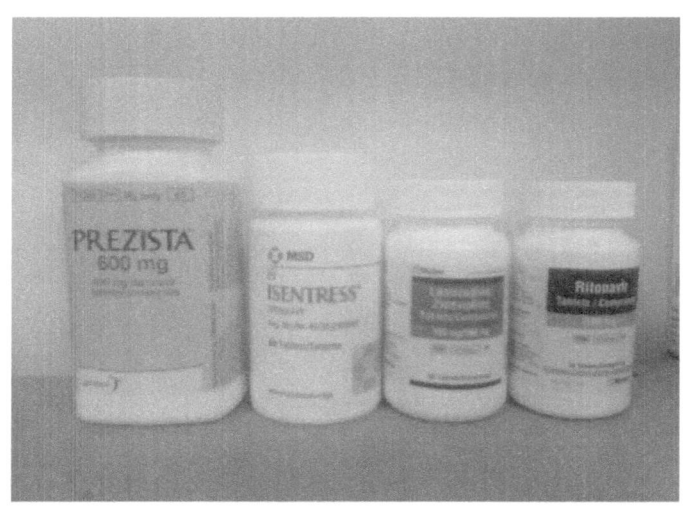

CHAPTER ONE

SOME NECESSARY CONCEPTS

Before the revision of the topics, specially the topic about the polypharmacy is my criteria that is very necessary to lead the reader in order to get information about some necessary concepts to understand better the disease and the treatment against the HIV virus and how does it works, and of course the phenomenon of the polypharmacy itself.

What is HIV?

The HIV or the Human Immunodeficiency Virus. This biologic agent is a lentivirus which is a subgroup of the retrovirus that causes the HIV infection. This infection leads the patient to the Acquired immunodeficiency syndrome a disease known as AIDS.

What is AIDS?

The conditions of the patient characterized by a progressive failure of the immune system and that allows the incubations of a lot of opportunistic infections in the human body and is the condition or the disease that we know as AIDS.

What is an antiretroviral drug ?.

An antiretroviral medicine is a drug destined to decrease the patient's total burden of the human immunodeficiency virus in the human blood, and to prevent the opportunistic diseases maintaining the function of the immune system.

The mean goal of this treatment is to reduce the quantity of the virus in the human blood. (The viraload).

There are several classes of drugs, which are usually used in combination, to treat HIV infection and which are broadly classified by the phase of the retrovirus life-cycle that the drug inhibits.

In this classification we can find the follow groups of medicines.

1)- Entry inhibitors

The entry inhibitors or the fusion inhibitors interfere with binding, fusion and entry of HIV-1 to the host cell by blocking one of several targets.

2)- Nucleoside reverse transcriptase inhibitors (NRTI)

This nucleoside reverse transcriptase inhibitors (NRTI) and nucleotide reverse transcriptase inhibitors (NtRTI) are nucleoside and nucleotide analogues which inhibit reverse transcription.

3)- Non-Nucleoside reverse transcriptase inhibitors (NNRTI)

The non-nucleoside reverse transcriptase inhibitors (NNRTI) inhibit reverse transcriptase by binding to an allosteric site of the enzyme; NNRTIs act as non-competitive inhibitors of reverse transcriptase.

4)-Integrase inhibitors

The integrase inhibitors and which are also known as the integrase nuclear strand transfer inhibitors or INSTIs, are drugs that inhibits the viral enzyme integrase, which are responsible for integration of the viral DNA into the DNA of the infected cell in the human body.

5)- Protease inhibitors

The protease inhibitors are drugs destined to block the viral protease enzyme necessary to produce mature virions upon budding from the host membrane.

What is HAART?

The HAART or the High Active Antiretroviral Therapy can be define as the use of multiple drugs that act against the HIV virus to stop its replication and to reduce the viraload in the human blood.

What is therapy ?

Therapy or treatment is define as the use of drugs for to treat any medical condition.

This drugs are selected taking into account the condition of the patient, the sensibility, the toxicity and another parameters.

What are the lines of treatment?

The lines of treatment refers to the types of regimens that we use in the patients taking into account the conditions of the patients specially the resistance to the treatment of any line.

What is the adherence ?

In the branch of the pharmacy, adherence is define as the degree in which a patient correctly follows the medical advices and concerning to the medicines, is closely related with the administration of the medication in the right dose and in the right time.

What are the side effects?

This concept represents the effects that appear as a consequence of the use of any drug and that appears just after the administration of the drug.

What is the adverse drug reaction?

An adverse drug reaction (ADR) is an injury that appears when the person take a medication and appear at the normal dose of the medication and just after the administration of this one.

What is the viraload?

To main goal of the treatment with the antiretroviral therapy is to get a very small viraload until to make it undetectable and to get at the same time a very high number of CD4 cells.

The viraload represents the quantity of the HIV virus in a blood drop.

What is de CD4?

The CD4 is a type of the T lymphocyte, some blood cells that constitutes the essential part of the immune system.

What is the treatment failure?

A pharmacological treatment use to fail when we don't use the drugs in the proper way and it leads to the apparition of some multi-drug resistant strains that can resist the presence and the effect of the medicine in the blood and to become in a very dominant genotypes in a short period of time.

Fixed-dose combinations

A fixed-dose-combination is the combinations of a lot of the antiretroviral drugs in the same formula bringing as a result an stander formula of several medicines. In this case we can show the emtricitabine +tenofovir disoproxil fumarate efavirenz. This the medicine known as Atripla. A first line antiretroviral drug.

What is PEP, Postexposure prophylaxis)?

This is the treatment that we offer to our patient just for to in direct contact with that blood of an infected person. This medication consists in TDF/FTC/ATV/r.

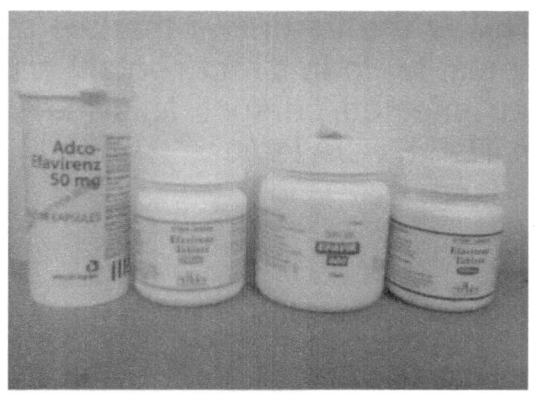

GENERAL RULES FOR THE CONSERVATION OF A MEDICATION

1. To maintain the medications in a dry and fresh place far from the heat and of the humidity.

2. To maintain the medications far from the children.

3. To keep the medicines in the refrigerator, placing the medicines in the drawers. The medicines must not be freeze.

4. To check you the container to find the maker's instructions on the conservation of this medication.

5. Never stores the medication near toxic substances.

RULES OF GOLD TO TAKE A CORRECT ADHERENCE TO THE MEDICATION

For to keep a correct adherence the patients must:

1 - To know their illness.

2 – To know their limitations.

3 - To know their medicines.

4 – To know the other names of their medications.

5 – To know to which medication is allergic or that the patient doesn't tolerate it.

6 – To communicate the doctor in the right time if is having improvement or not.

7 – To be sincere with the doctor.

8 – To take the medicine in the correct time and every day at the same time without to miss any dose.

9-Never leave a medication within reach of the children.

BASIC ORIENTATIONS TO THE PATIENT FOR THE CORRECT USE OF THE ANTIRETROVIRAL DRUGS

1. In the first appointment you must tell to your doctor if you are allergic to any medicine.
2. Take the medicine every day at the same time.
3. Take the medicine just as the doctor says.
4. Never give the medicine to another person.
5. Keep the medicine far from the children.
6. Never drink alcohol during the treatment.
7. Take the medicine near the food and never with the stomach empty, avoid the gastritis and esophagitis.
8. Come to see your doctor in the right follow up date.
9. Never miss a dose.
10. If you miss a dose please tell that to the doctor and to the pharmacist.
11. Come to the follow up date with the remaining tablets.
12. Take the medicine with a glass of water.
13. If you are pregnant and you are under treatment with antiretroviral therapy you must take your medicines

with juice of fruits for to supply your body of vitamins.
14. Never take a medicine without the orientation or prescriptions of the physician.
15. You must communicate to the doctor about any side effect that you experience.
16. Store the medicines in a safe and dry place.
17. In every appointment tell to your doctor about any improvement in your status.

CHAPTER TWO

SOME ANTIRETROVIRAL DRUGS ITS ABBREVIATIONS AND SIDE EFFECTS

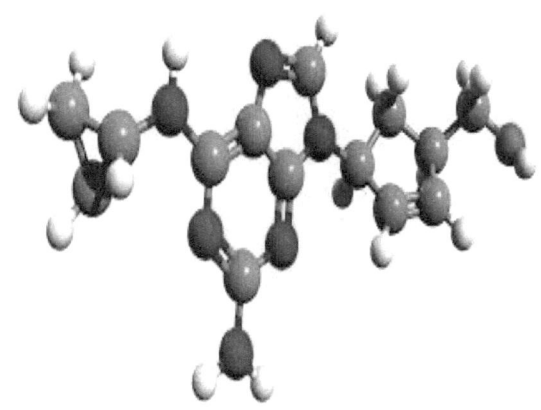

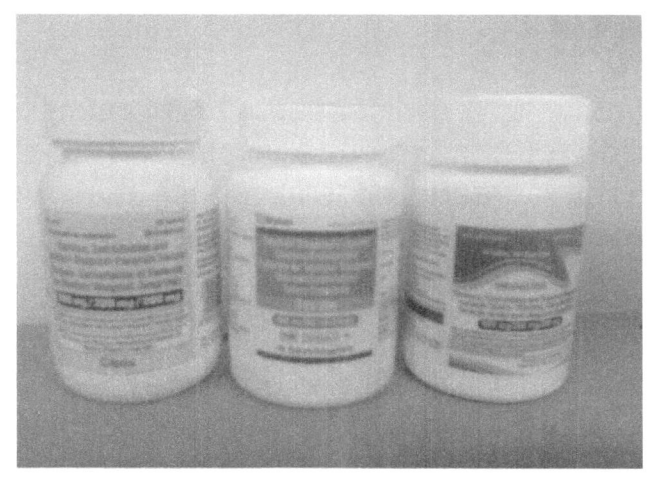

What is a antiretroviral drug ?.

An antiretroviral medicine is a drug destined to decrease the patient's total burden of the human immunodeficiency virus in the human blood, and to prevent the opportunistic diseases maintaining the function of the immune system. The mean goal of this treatment is to reduce the quantity of the virus in the human blood. (The viraload).

There are several classes of drugs, which are usually used in combination, to treat HIV infection and which are broadly classified by the phase of the retrovirus life-cycle that the drug inhibits.

In this classification we can find the follow groups of medicines.

Nucleoside/Nucleotide Reverse Transcriptase Inhibitors (NRTIs)

Some examples of this group of the antiretroviral medicines are:

Antiretroviral drug   Abbreviation

- Abacavir   ABC
- Didanosine   DDI
- Emtricitabine   FTC
- Lamivudine   3TC
- Stavudine   D4T
- Tenofovir   TDF
- Zidovudine   AZT

Non-nucleoside Reverse Transcriptase Inhibitors (NNRTIs)

Some examples of this group of the antiretroviral medicines are:

Antiretroviral drug   Abbreviation

- Delavirdine   DLV
- Efavirenz   EFV
- Etravirine   ETR
- Nevirapine   NVP
- Rilpivirine   RPV

Protease Inhibitors

Some examples of this group of the antiretroviral medicines are:

Antiretroviral drug   Abbreviation

The antiretroviral drugs use to have an abbreviation of its names, and most of the physicians use to prescribe these abbreviations in the passport of the patients.

I must say that idea is not good because sometimes the patients does not check the containers and when they do it the name in the container of the medicine does not match with the prescription made by the physician, and it can develop the phenomenon of nom-adherence to the treatment and it use to happen in persons with low cultural level. Some examples are:

- Amprenavir.
- Atazanavir   ATV
- Darunavir   DRV
- Fosamprenavir   FPV
- Indinavir   IDV
- Lopinavir/ Ritonavir LPV/r
- Nelfinavir   NFV
- Ritonavir   RTV
- Saquinavir   SQV

- Tipranavir   TPV
- Bictegravir   BIC
- Dolutegravir   DTG
- Elvitegravir   EVG
- Raltegravir   RAL

Fixed-Dose Combinations

Some examples of the medicines that was fixed in some fix dose combinations and its abbreviations are:

- Abacavir + dolutegravir + lamivudine, or ABC/DTG/3TC (Triumeq)
- Abacavir + lamivudine, or ABC/3TC (Epzicom)
- Abacavir + lamivudine + zidovudine, or ABC/3TC/ZDV (Trizivir)
- Atazanavir + cobicistat, or ATV/c (Evotaz)
- Atazanavir + cobicistat, or ATV/c (Evotaz)
- Bictegravir + emtricitabine + tenofovir alafenamide, or BIC/FTC/TAF (Biktarvy)
- Dolutegravir + rilpivirine, or DTG/RPV (Juluca)
- Durunavir + cobicistat, or DRV/c (Prezcobix)
- Efavirenz + emtricitabine + tenofovir, or EFV/FTC/TDF (Atripla)
- Elvitegravir + cobicistat + emtricitabine + tenofovir, or EVG/c/FTC/TAF (Genvoya)
- Elvitegravir + cobicistat + emtricitabine + tenofovir, or

EVG/COBI/FTC/TDF or ECF/TDF (Stribild)
- Emtricitabine + rilpivirine + tenofovir, or FTC/RPV/TAF (Odefsey)
- Emtricitabine + rilpivirine + tenofovir, or FTC/RPV/TDF (Complera)
- Emtricitabine + tenofovir, or TAF/FTC (Descovy)
- Emtricitabine + tenofovir, or TDF/FTC (Truvada)
- Lamivudine + zidovudine, or 3TC/ZDV (Combivir)

SOME ANTIRETROVIRAL MEDICINES AND ITS SIDE EFFECTS

Is well known that the antiretroviral medicines are having some side effects that constitute a characteristic of this pharmacologic group of medicines specially the Nephrotoxicity, the gynecomastia and the psychosis, and the more representative drugs are the tenofovir disoproxil or TDF and the Efaverens or EFV.

In this small chapter I want to show just some of these medicines and their general side effects in the patients that are living with HIV/AIDS.

Together with the name and the abbreviations the reader can appreciate the chemical structure of these medicines.

I)- LOPINAVIR /RITONAVIR LPV

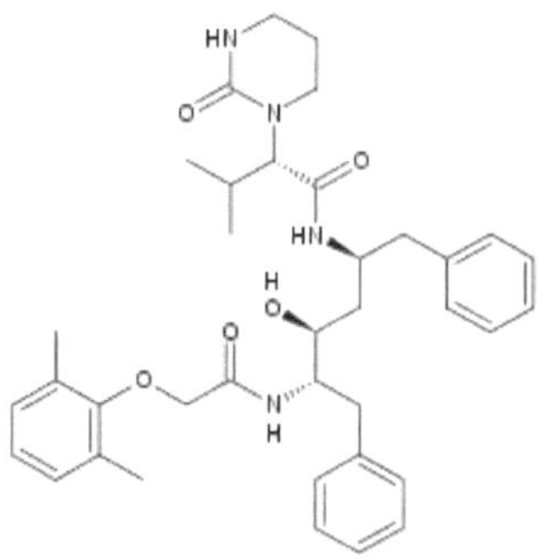

Picture # 1. Chemical structure of LOPINAVIR.

Side effect: The Diarrhea, the headache, nausea,, also the vomiting and, drowsiness as the dizziness, a bad taste in the mouth of the patient and even the trouble sleeping are normal side effect of this drug..

II)-RITONAVIR Rit

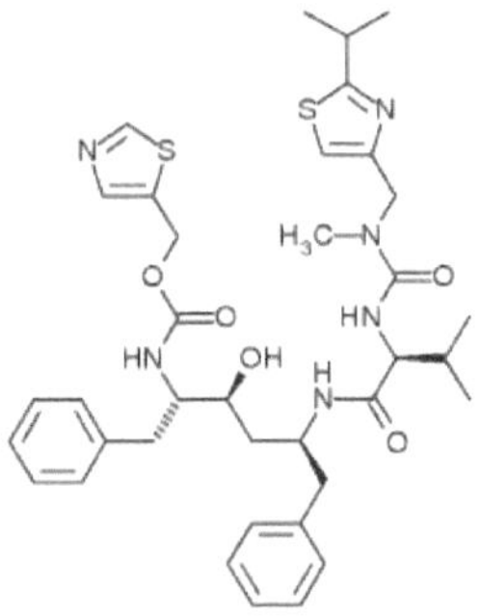

Picture # 2. Chemical structure of RITONAVIR.

Side effect: Some of the side effects of this drug are the inflammation of the pancreas which is also known as pancreatitis, problems in the rhythm of the hart, severe allergic reactions and liver problems among others.

III)- ABACADIR ABC

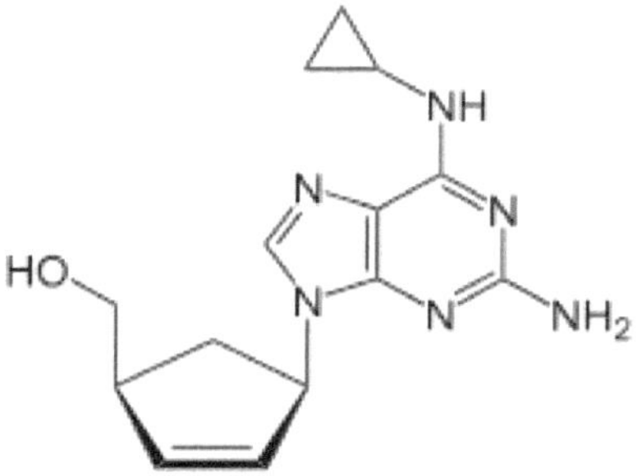

Picture # 3. Chemical structure of ABACADIR.

side effects: The side effects of the abacadir are, the vomiting, the fever, the trouble sleeping and the weakness sensation in the body. The lactic acidosis and the damage in the liver can appear as severe side effects also.

IV)- TENOFOVIR DISOPROXIL TDF

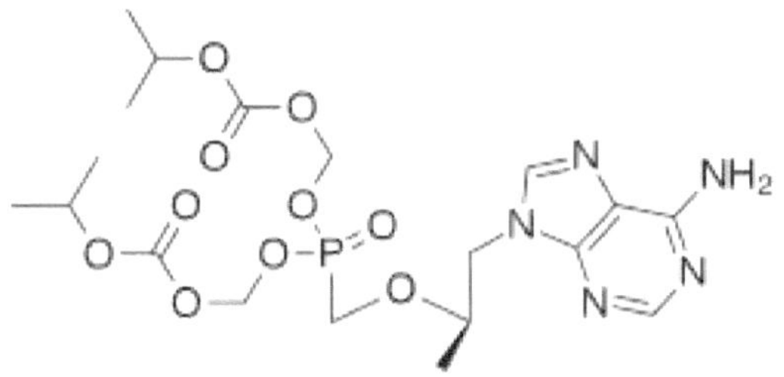

Picture # 4. Chemical structure of TENOFOVIR DISOPROXIL.

Side effects: In the case of the tenofovir they are the nausea, the rash in the skin, the diarrhea, headache, pain, depression, and weakness. It can bring also enlarged liver.

VI)- ENTRICITABINE FTC

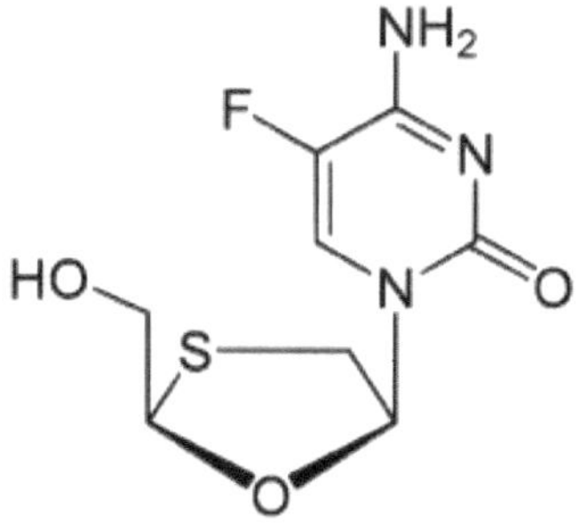

Picture # 5. Chemical structure of ETRICITABINE.

Side effects: Some side effects of emtricitabine are the lactic acidosis and serious liver problems.

VI)-EFAVERENS EFV.

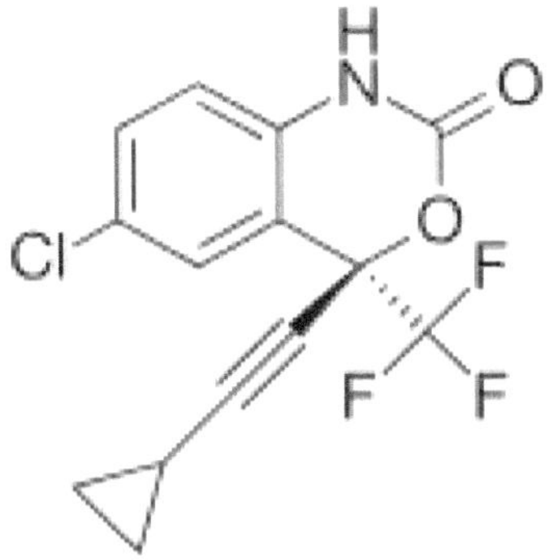

Picture # 6. Chemical structure of the EFAVERENS.

Side effects: The side effect of efaverens are the rash in the skin, the nausea, headache and weakness. In some patients it can brings the Stevens-Johnson syndrome

VII)- Rilpivirine

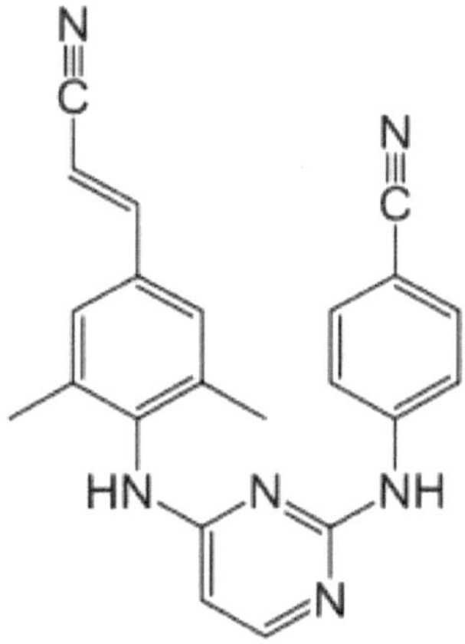

Picture # 7. Chemical structure of RILPIVIRINE .

Side effect: the rash in the skin, the depression and the trouble Sleeping are side effects of this drug.

VIII)-Elvitegravir EVG.

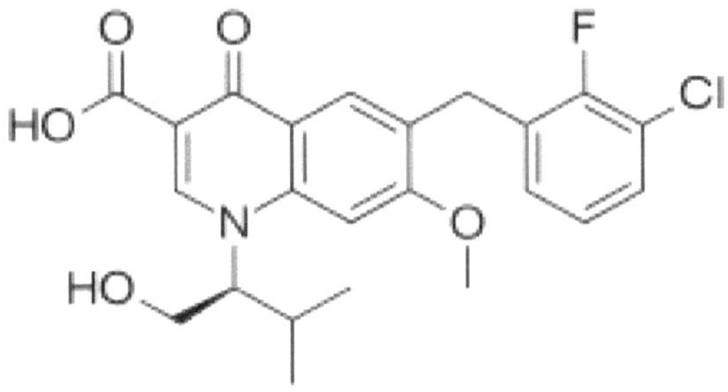

Picture # 8. Chemical structure of ELVITRGRAVIR.

Side effect: One of the serious side effects of this drug is the **inflammatory syndrome (IRIS and also the** diarrhea which is the common one.

IX)- Dolutegravir DTG.

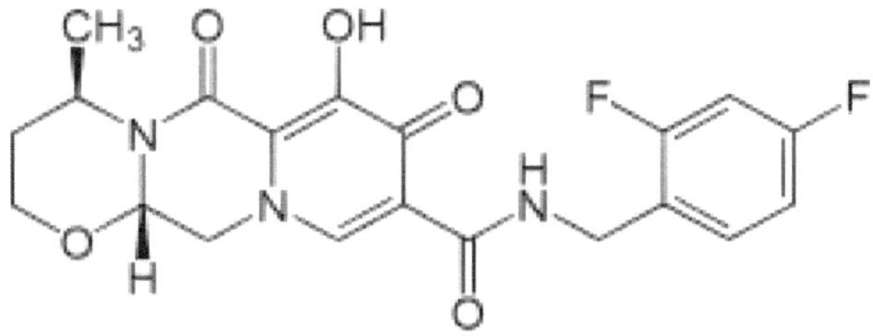

Picture # 9. Chemical structure of DOLUTEGRAVIR.

Side effects: The trouble sleeping, the weakness, the liver problems and the increase of the sugar level in the human blood are side effects of the dolutegravir.

X)-ATAZANAVIR ATV/r

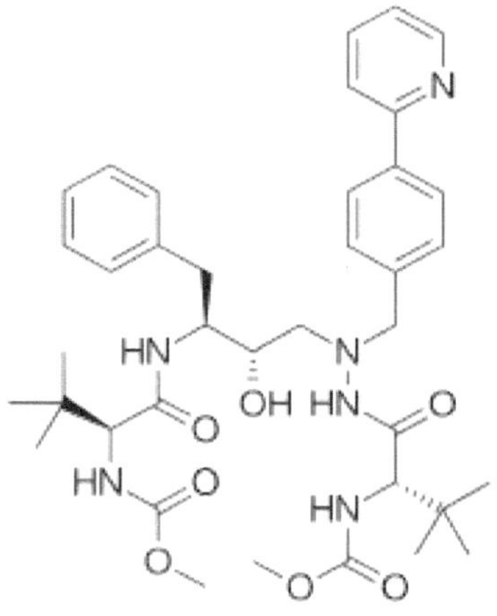

Picture # 10. Chemical structure of ATAZANAVIR.

Side effect: The Headache, nausea and the yellowish skin with the abdominal pain are side effect of this drug.

XI)-DURANAVIR DRV.

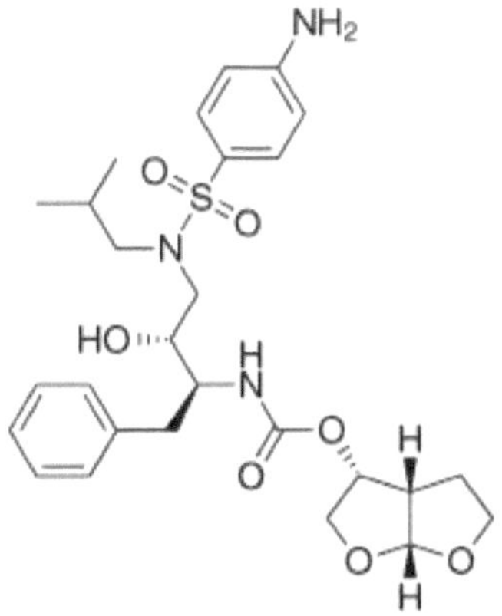

Picture # 11. Chemical structure of DURANAVIR.

Side effects: Some of the side effect of this drug are the diarrhea, the nausea, the headache and the toxic epidermal necrolysis, a very serious disease very similar to the Stevens-Johnson syndrome where the skin of the patient looks like a burned skin.

XII)-RETALGRAVIR RAL.

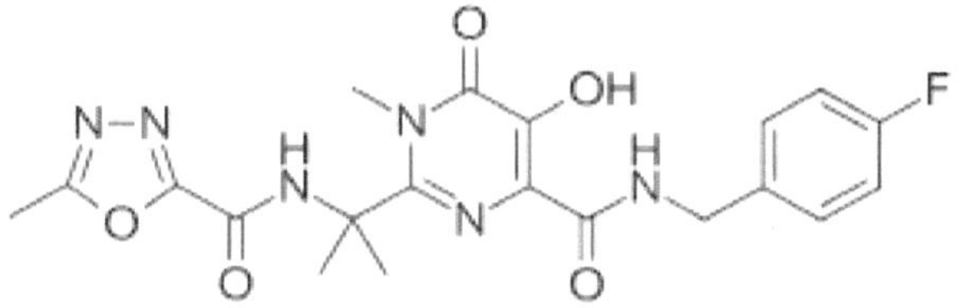

Picture # 12. Chemical structure of DURANAVIR.

Side effects: the side effects of this drug include the trouble sleeping, the weakness also the Stevens-Johnson syndrome.

XIII)-Niveripine NVP.

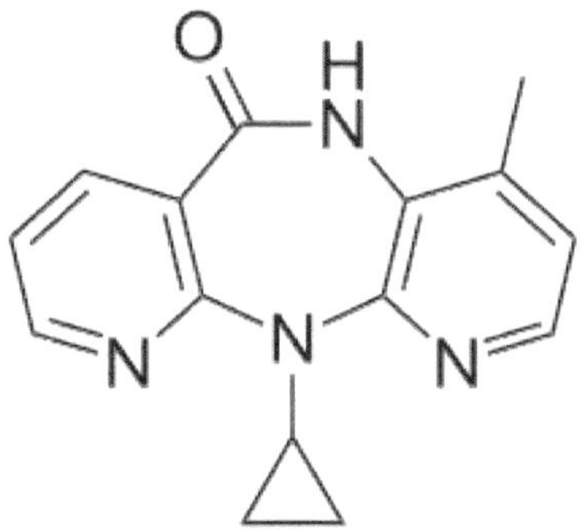

Picture # 13. Chemical structure of Niveripine.

Side effects: The rash in the skin, the, headache, nausea, feeling tired, and liver problems, includes the side effects of this medicine.

XIV)-STAVUDINE D4T.

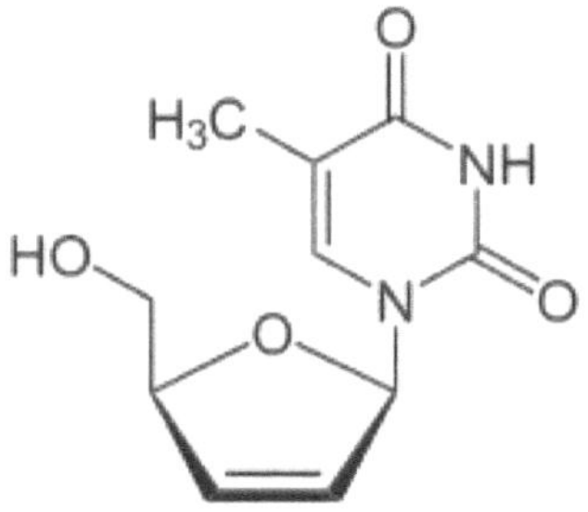

Picture # 14. Chemical structure of STAVUDINE.

Side effects: Some side effects of this drug are the headache, the diarrhea, the vomiting, and the rash, in the skin.

XV)- DADOSINE DDI.

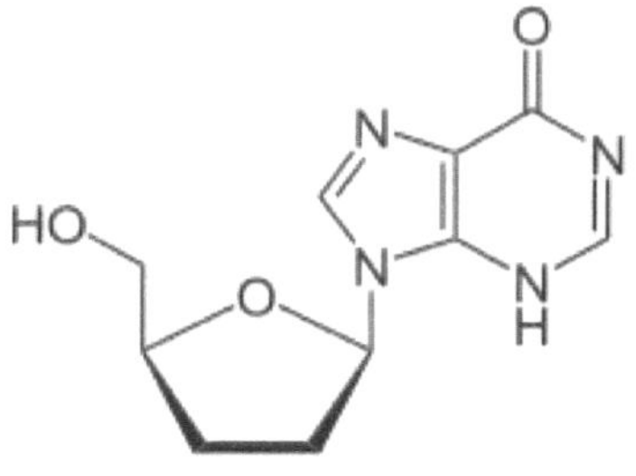

Picture # 15. Chemical structure of Didanosine.

Side effects: The side effects of the didanosine are the nausea, the stomachache the fever, the itching, and the rash in the skin.

XVI)-LAMIVUDINE 3TC

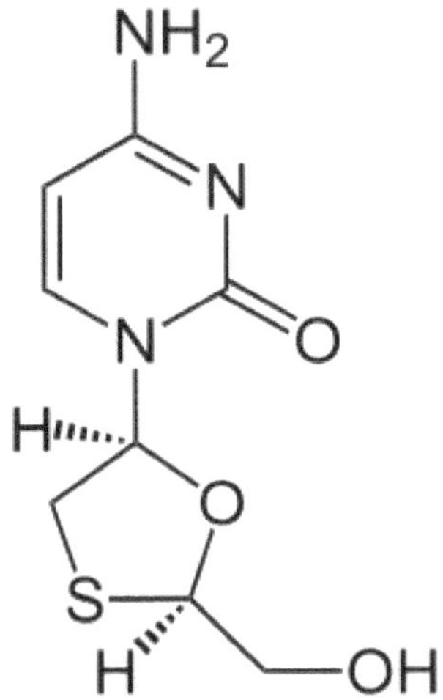

Picture # 16. Chemical structure of Lamivudine

Side effect: Some side effects of lamivudine the lactic acidosis and the severe liver problems and the inflammation in the pancreas, a disease that we know as pancreatitis.

XVII)-ZIDOVUDINE

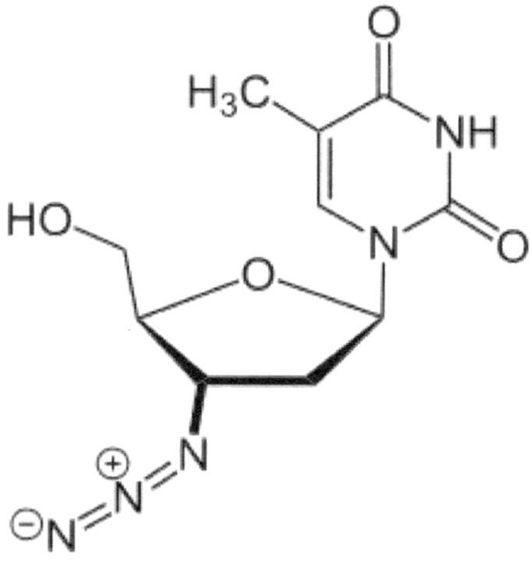

Picture # 17. Chemical structure of Zidovudine

Side effects: Some side effects of zidovudine are the lactic acidosis and problems in the liver severe anemia (neutropenia). and myopathy.

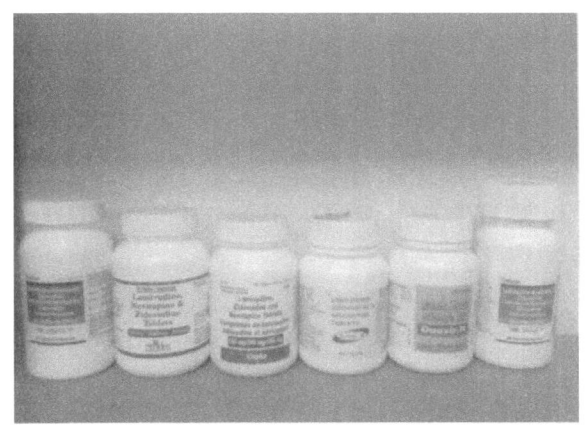

CHAPTER TWO

POLYPHARMACY

(A simple explanation about the treatment with ARV)

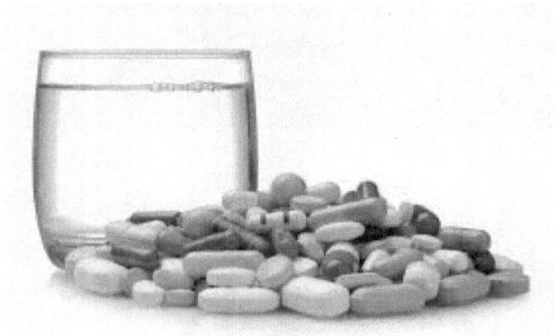

CHAPTER TWO

POLYPHARMACY

The polypharmacy has been defined as the use of multiple medications for the treatment of a patient's medical conditions. This criteria suggests that the patient is using more medication than the quantity of the medications that has been indicated by the physician and also that the number of medicines taken by a patient that can constitutes polypharmacy has not been defined.

Which are the causes of the polypharmacy?

In order to define the causes of the polypharmacy we must talk about the fellow criteria.

1. The medical conditions of the patient.

(The increase of the negative medical conditions produces an increase in the number of the medications to treat each condition).

2. The hospitalization of the patient.

(A new risk (*infection*) increase the use of the preventive medication).

3. The number of the prescriptors.

(Multiple doctors are prescribing medications for the same patient. Once a patient starts a medication, it is never discontinued).

4. Change of the treatment.

(Doctors changes from one medication to another within the same therapeutic class; but the patient doesn't stop taking the first medication).

5. The incidence of the regimen (some regimes have more medicines than the others. (Because of the combination).

Polypharmacy and the RDP (related drugs problems)

The polypharmacy can bring itself some related drugs problems in the treatment of the patients who are living with HIV virus, among them we can find:

1. Unnecessary and/or inappropriate medication prescribing
2. Increased risk for drug interactions and adverse drug reactions
3. Non adherence
4. Increased overall drug expenditures.
5. Decisions by the patients (AUTO-ABANDOM or AUTO-MEDICATION (*self-medication*)).
6. The problem of to treat *side effects* with a new medicines which are having also *side effects.*
7. The terrible problem of to treat side effects with one or more drugs like symptoms of one diseases by mistake when it is really a side effect.

Well practice of the prescription for to avoid the polypharmacy

The well practice of the prescription can avoid the polypharmacy in some patients taking into account that some of our patients can lies to the doctor concerning to the adherence to the treatment and can lies also concerning to the idea if the patients are taking any medicine by theirs own ways.

1. Maintain an accurate medication and medical history.
2. Link each prescribed medication to a disease state.
3. Identify medications that are treating side effects.
4. Initiate interventions to ensure adherence.
5. Reconcile medications upon discharge from hospital

Now in this topic we will represent a normal treatment to and adult patient who is living with HIV virus. In this example the patient starts from the first line going throw the pharmacological arsenal taking into account of course the clinical condition of the patient concerning to the resistance to the first line or second line and if the patient was having any contact with patients who are living with TB, that is to say; tuberculosis.

In this example we can observe the evolution of the patient from the PEP (post exposure prophylaxis for HIV) to the third line of the treatment.

We can observe how the quantity of the medicines and the risk can increase continuously throw the time.

Antiretroviral therapy for adults patients who are in PEP

I)-TDF/FTC/ ATV/r for 28 DAYS

In this case the patient takes 2 tablets daily of 4 different medicines.

In this case the patient can just experience some side effects like stomachache because is starting a new medicine and sometimes the patients use to take the tablet in the morning with the stomach empty but there are not side effect or toxicity like for to put in danger the patient's life.

ANTIRETROVIRAL THERAPY FOR ADULTS PATIENTS WHO ARE LIVING WITH HIV. FIRST LINE

The prescriptons for the adult patient who is living with HIV.

Treatment in first line. (just for to treat Antiretroviral Therapy for Adults patients who are living with HIV. FIRST LINE HIV and prevention against fungal infection):

1. TDF/FTC/EFV 1 tab. OD. Night time.
2. MTV 1 tab. OD. In the morning
3. CTX 2 tab. OD. At night time.

In this case the patient takes 4 tablets daily of 5 different medicines.

Treatment in first line. (just for to treat HIV and prevention against fungal infection):

Same treatment for the same patent in first line if the patient is feeling pain

1) TDF/FTC/EFV 1 tab. OD. Night time.

2) MTV 1 tab. OD. In the morning

3) CTX 2 tab. OD. At night time.

4) PANADO 500mg. 2 tab. TDS. (3 times daily).

In this case the patient takes 10 tablets daily of 6 different medicines.

Same treatment for the same patent in first line if the patient is feeling pain and articular pain.

Treatment in first line. (just for to treat HIV and prevention against fungal infection):

1) TDF/FTC/EFV 1 tab. OD. Nigth time.

2) MTV 1 tab. OD. In the morning

3) CTX 2 tab. OD. At night time.

4) PANADO 500mg. 2 tab. TDS. (3 times daily).

5) Methylsalicilate ointment apply 2 times daily.

In this case the patient takes 10 tablets daily and apply 1 ointment 2 times daily (BD) of 7 different medicines.

Same treatment for the same patent in first line if the patient is feeling pain and articular pain and the patient is in prophylaxis of TB.

Treatment in first line. (just for to treat HIV and prevention against fungal infection):

1) TDF/FTC/EFV 1 tab. OD. Nigth time.

2) MTV 1 tab. OD. In the morning

3) CTX 2 tab. OD. At night time.

4) PANADO 500mg. 2 tab. TDS. (3 times daily).

5) Methylsalicilate ointment apply 2 times daily.

6) Isoniazid (INH) 300 mg 1 tablet OD. In the morning.

7) Piridoxine 25 mg. 1 tablet OD. In the morning.

In this case the patient takes 12 tablets daily and apply 1 ointment 2 times daily of 9 different medicines.

Antiretroviral Therapy for Adults patients who are living with HIV and not tolerate the EFAVERENZ. Technically in FIRST LINE.

The prescriptions for the adult patient who is living with HIV.

Treatment in second line. (just for to treat HIV and prevention against fungal infection):

1. TDF/3TC/AZT/LPV/r
2. TDF/3TC 300 mg/ 150 mg 1 tab. OD. Night time.
3. AZT 300 mg 1 tab. BD (1 tab in the morning/ 1 tab. In the night)
4. LPV/r 200 mg/ 100 mg. 2 tab. BD (2 tab in the morning/ 2 tab. In the night).
5. MTV 1 tab. OD. In the morning
6. CTX 2 tab. OD. At night time.

In this case the patient takes 9 tablets daily of 6 different medicines.

Same treatment for the same patient in first line if the patient is felling pain.

Treatment in second line. (Just for to treat HIV and prevention against fungal infection):

1. TDF/3TC/AZT/LPV/r
2. TDF/3TC 300 mg/ 150 mg 1 tab. OD. Nigth time.
3. AZT 300 mg 1 tab. BD (1 tab in the morning/ 1 tab. In the night)
4. LPV/r 200 mg/ 100 mg. 2 tab. BD (2 tab in the morning/ 2 tab. In the night).
5. MTV 1 tab. OD. In the morning
6. CTX 2 tab. OD. At night time.
7. PANADO 500 mg 2 tab. TDS. (3 times per day).

In this case the patient takes 15 tablets daily from 7 different medicines.

Same treatment for the same patient in first line if the patient is felling pain and articular pain.

Treatment in second line. (just for to treat HIV and prevention against fungal infection):

1. TDF/3TC/AZT/LPV/r
2. TDF/3TC 300 mg/ 150 mg 1 tab. OD. Nigth time.
3. AZT 300 mg 1 tab. BD (1 tab in the morning/ 1 tab. In the night)
4. LPV/r 200 mg/ 100 mg. 2 tab. BD (2 tab in the morning/ 2 tab. In the night).
5. MTV 1 tab. OD. In the morning
6. CTX 2 tab. OD. At night time.
7. PANADO 500 mg 2 tab. TDS. (3 times per day).
8. Methylsalicilate ointment. Apply 2 times per day.

In this case the patient takes 15 tablets daily and apply 1 ointment 2 times daily and using 8 different medicines.

Same treatment for the same patient in first line if the patient is felling pain and articular pain and the patient is in prophylaxis of TB.

Treatment in second line. (just for to treat HIV and prevention against fungal infection):

1. TDF/3TC/AZT/LPV/r
2. TDF/3TC 300 mg/ 150 mg 1 tab. OD. Nigth time.
3. AZT 300 mg 1 tab. BD (1 tab in the morning/ 1 tab. In the night)
4. LPV/r 200 mg/ 100 mg. 2 tab. BD (2 tab in the morning/ 2 tab. In the night).
5. MTV 1 tab. OD. In the morning
6. CTX 2 tab. OD. At night time.
7. PANADO 500 mg 2 tab. TDS. (3 times per day).
8. Methylsalicilate ointment . Apply 2 times per day.
9. ISONIAZID (INH) 300 mg. 1 tab. OD. In the morning.
10. PIRIDOXINE 25 mg. 1 tab. OD. In the morning.

In this case the patient takes 17 tablets daily and apply 1 ointment 2 times daily of 10 different medicines.

Some factors that can predispose individuals to the adverse effects of th antiretrovirals medicines

- Concomitant use of medications with overlapping and additive toxicities
- Comorbid conditions that increase the risk of or exacerbate adverse effects (,or example the alcoholism or co-infection with viral hepatitis may increase the risk of hepatotoxicity; psychiatric disorders may be exacerbated by efavirenz [EFV]- and, infrequently, by integrase strand transfer inhibitor [INSTI]-related CNS toxicities; and borderline or mild renal dysfunction increases the risk of nephrotoxicity from tenofovir disoproxil fumarate [TDF])
- Drug-drug interactions that may increase toxicities of ARV drugs or concomitant medications
- Genetic factors that predispose patients to abacavir (ABC) hypersensitivity reaction, EFV neuropsychiatric toxicity, and atazanavir (ATV)-associated hyperbilirubinemia.

Some of the consecuences of the polypharmacy

The polypharmacy in the patients who are living with HIV can bring and increase the possibilities of an adverse drug reactions. It can produces an increase of the possibility of the interactions between the medications, the increase of the toxicity of the medicines and among other things; the increase of the damage in the aim organs with takes part in the metabolism of these drugs, An elevation in the possibility of the apparition of more than one side effects of different medicines at the same time witch can injure the health of the patient and an increasing in the possibility of toxicity if we treat and adverse drugs reaction with a medicine witch can produce another side effect or another adverse drug reaction and this last one is very important because it can be very dangerous for the patient's life.

Discussion

Taking into account the appreciation of the previous prescriptions we can observe how the polypharmacy take part itself in the patients how are living with HIV, in this case for the adult patients which are having an standard treatment for to reduce the multiplication of the virus and for to prevent the apparition of 2 opportunist diseases. In the previous treatment we can see how the risk of the interactions between medicines increase itself while we are prescribing the superior regimen because the patient reach the other regimen sometimes because of the resistance of the virus which means that the immunologic system is weak and therefore the apparition of the opportunists diseases We can observe that when we include a new medicine in the treatment, the risk of the side effects increase itself in a proportional relation with the increase of the therapy and it can justify that the polypharmacy is very closely from the Related Drugs Problems in the patient and that they can produce it.

We can observe that the ARV (antiretroviral) therapy is a polypharmacy itself taking into account the quantity of medication.

SOME CONTROVERSIAL SITUATIONS

Undetectable patients and prophylaxis with cotromazole 480 mg

In this discussion we can see that some of our patients are undetectable, so, if the immune system is having a good level, the CD4 is very high and the viraload is very low; then: Why should we maintain the treatment of prophylaxis for fungal infection when the patient does not need it or the patient is not having symptoms of the disease.

Patient with contact with another patient who is having tuberculosis as a definitive diagnosis for more than three month and the patient does not shows any symptom of the disease.

In this case we can say that this patient is taking Izoniazid increasing the polypharmacy and the possibilities of side effects

In both cases the better advice is to check the medical condition of the patient and to confirm the diagnosis before to prescribe the medicines.

Conclusions

1- We can affirm that the polypharmacy is related to the regimen of the treatment for the patient who is living with HIV and that is very related to the apparition of the side effect, the interactions between the drugs .

2-We can see that the concept of polypharmacy is very controversial and that it depends of some factors as the quantity of drugs, the well practice of the prescription and the auto-medication (self-medication).

Recommendations

1- To exert the well practice of the prescription of the medicines taking into account that we must treat patients no diseases.

2- To know the characteristics of the patient and his adherence to the treatment and to check this adherences in every appointment.

3- To prescribe the medicines for to avoid the disease not for to give pleasure to the patient.

4- To know the concept of the polypharmacy and its applications.

CHAPTER THREE
SELF-MEDICATION AND THE TOXICITY OF THE PARACETAMOL

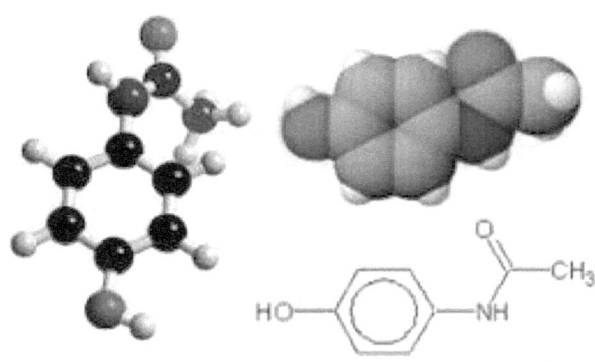

THE TOXICITY OF THE PARACETAMOL

Paracetamol, also known as *acetaminophen, panado, tylenol,* is a NSAIDs (Nom Steroidal Anti-inflammatory Drugs), which is used to treat pain and fever, especially for the treatment of the pain for example in the case of the moderate pain and for more severe pain such as cancer pain and after surgery and its effects last between two and four hours.

This drug is safe when we use it in the recommended doses.

This drug can produce a serious skin rashes but it is very rare but when we use too high doses it can result in liver failure.

The paracetamol is a drug that we can use under the criteria that is very safe during pregnancy and during the breastfeeding also.

In the case that we treat a patient with a liver disease; even like that is useful but it should be taken in lower doses.

The paracetamol is classified as a mild analgesic and is good to say that It does not have significant anti-inflammatory activity.

The World Health Organization (WHO) recommends that paracetamol be used to treat fever in children only if their temperature is greater than 38.5 °C.

Pharmacokinetic

After oral administration it is rapidly absorbed by the gastrointestinal tract; its volume of distribution is roughly 50 L.

The concentration in serum after a typical dose of paracetamol usually peaks below 30 µg/ml, which equals 200 µmol/L. After 4 hours the concentration is usually less than 10 µg/mL, which equals 66 µmol/L.

Paracetamol is metabolized primarily in the liver, into toxic and non-toxic products. Three metabolic pathways are notable:

1- Glucuronidation (45-55%), by UGT1A1 and UGT1A6.
2- Sulfation (sulfate conjugation) (20–30%) by SULT1A1.

3- *N*-hydroxylation and dehydration, then GSH conjugation, (less than 15%).

The hepatic cytochrome P450 enzyme system metabolizes paracetamol, forming a minor yet significant alkylating metabolite known as NAPQI (*N*-acetyl-*p*-benzoquinone imine) (also known as *N*-acetylimidoquinone). NAPQI is then irreversibly conjugated with the sulfhydryl groups of glutathione.

All three pathways yield final products that are inactive, non-toxic, and eventually excreted by the kidneys. In the third pathway, however, the intermediate product NAPQI is toxic. NAPQI is primarily responsible for the toxic effects of paracetamol.

The toxicity

The toxicity of acetaminophen is closely linked to its metabolism. With therapeutic dosing, acetaminophen is predominantly metabolized by conjugation with sulfate and glucuronide.

The NAPQI that is not detoxified may bind to hepatocytes and produce cellular necrosis

There is also a very controversial situation because sometimes we don't indicate a minimum dose for toxicity, but we find a relation between the prolongation of the half-life of acetaminophen and the liver toxicity.

THE SELF MEDICATION PROBLEMS

1. No medical prescription.
2. No correct dosage of the medicine.
3. No weight taken to the patient for to relate the dose with the patient.
4. No knowledge of the clinical situation of the patient.
5. No discussion of the behavior of the patient with the Parents.
6. The doctor doesn't see the patient.
7. Sometimes the person who gets the medicine is not the person where the child is staying.
8. Wrong recommendation of the medicine.
9. There is not dispensation of the medicine and therefore there is not any orientation to the patient about the use of the medicine.
10. There is not following of the treatment by the physician.

Situation at the pharmacy

1- The patient asks for the medicine instead to see the doctor.
2- The patient change the treatment from panado to brufen or to any other NSAIDs without to see the doctor.
3- The patient refuse the words of the pharmacist about to take the orientations concerning to this medicine.
4- The several languages of the patents and the ignorance make a wall between the patient and pharmacist.

Comercial situation

1- The big availability out of the state hospital. (Private sector, shops, malls,) at low price.

Why paracetamol should be take only under medical prescription

1-Liver damage

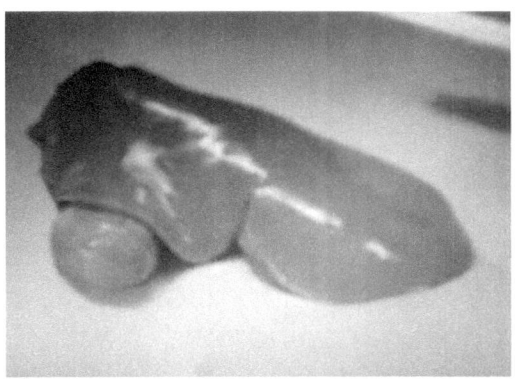

Picture # 4. It represents a damage liver.

The acute overdoses of paracetamol can cause potentially fatal liver damage. Paracetamol is metabolized by the liver and is hepatotoxic; side effects are multiplied when combined with alcoholic drinks, and are very likely in chronic alcoholics or patients with liver damage.

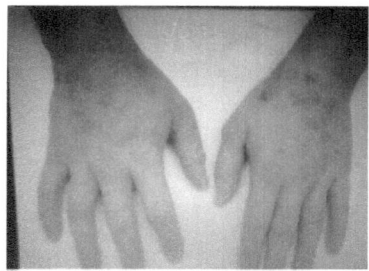

Picture # 5. This picture represents a patient with rash cutaneous in both hands.

It stated that the drug could cause rare, and possibly fatal, skin reactions, such as Stevens–Johnson syndrome and toxic epidermal necrolysis.

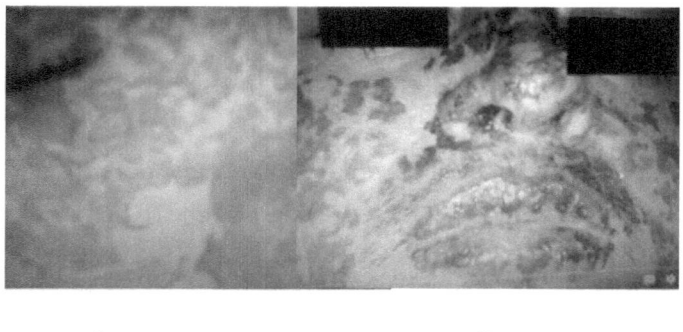

A   B

Picture # 6. A and B represents a patients with Stevens–Johnson syndrome.

ORIENTATIONS FOR THE CORRECT USE OF THE PARACETAMOL

1. Take this medicine just under medical prescription.
2. Follow the treatment step by step just as the pharmacist say.
3. Read the leaflet of your medicine.
4. Don't take the advice of any other person just the advice of the physician and the pharmacist.
5. Don't recommend your medicine to any other person.
6. Don't drink any other Nom Steroidal Anti-inflammatory Drug during the treatment with paracetamol.
7. Don't drink alcohol during the treatment.
8. If you feel something like rash cutaneous, eruption in the skin or any other symptoms stop the treatment immediately and go to see your doctor or pharmacist again.
9. Keep this medicine very far from the sight and the reach of children.
10. Store this medicine in a dry and secure place.
11. Take your medicine every day at the same time.

12. If you vomit during the treatment you must check.. If you find the whole tablet then after thirty minutes you can drink another tablet, otherwise if you don't find the whole tablet don't drink another one.

13. If you miss a dose the next day don't drink two doses just the dose indicated by the physician.

14. Keep your medicine in the correct container and never mix your tablet with another one.

15. If you are going to travel, travel always with your medicine.

A revision of the side effects of the antiretroviral therapy

Perhaps the treatment with antiretroviral therapy is the most complicated treatment for a disease, taking into account the risk of the sides effects of this medication which is always considerate a treatment in polypharmacy for each patient.

The antiretroviral therapy is a brand of 3 of 4 medicines in a combination where each one of them are having a purpose and where the goal of the treatment is impossible without this combination, and for that reason the risk of the sides effects increase in this treatment itself.

The medication of the patient is having two branch. Number one: The basic treatment (ARVs) and Number two: Complementary treatment (Medicines for to avoid the opportunists diseases) which increase the quantity of the medicines and the risk of the sides effects.

Some factors that can predispose individuals to adverse effects or side effects of the ARV medications

Some of the factors that can predispose our patients to the side effects of the medicines includes the concomitant use of medications, the comorbid in the clinical conditions of the patients that can increase the risk or to become the patient more sensible to the side effects of the antiretroviral drugs such as the alcoholism or the co-infection with viral hepatitis which can brings a big risk of hepatotoxicity and psychiatric disorders witch can be exacerbated by efaverenz among others examples. Also the Drug-drug interactions increase toxicities during the treatment specially when we treat our patients with concomitant medications. In other hand the genetic factors can predispose the patients to a hypersensitivity reaction to abacavir (ABC).

ABBREVIATIONS

ABC- Abacadir

AIDS- Adquire Inmunodeficense Syndromen

ARV- Antiretroviral

ARVs- Antiretrovirals

ATV/r- Atazanavir

AZT- Zidovudine

BD- Twice daily

CNS-Central Nervous System

COX- Cyclooxygenase, its official name Is prostaglandin endoperoxide synthase (PTGS).

COX-2-Cyclooxygenase-2. Its official name is (Prostaglandin Synthase-2).

CTX-Cotrimoxazole

CYPZE1- Is a member of the cytochrome P450 family of oxidizing enzymes.

CYP3A4- Is a member of the cytochrome P450 family of oxidizing enzymes.

DNA- Deoxyribonucleic acid.

DLT-Dolutegravir

EFV-Efaverenz

FTC- Emtricitabine, an antiretroviral drug used to treat HIV.

GSH-Growth hormone secretagogue.

HIV-Human Inmunodeficence Virus

INSTI- Integrase Strand Transfer inhibitors.

INH-Izoniazide

LPV/r-Lopinavir/Ritonavir

MVT-Multivitamine

N- Nytrogen

NSAIDs-NomSteroidal antiinflamatory drugs

NtRTI- Nucleotide reverse transcriptase inhibitors.

NNRT- Nucleoside reverse transcriptase

NNRT- Non-nucleoside reverse transcriptase

NNRTI- Non-nucleoside reverse transcriptase inhibitors

NVP-Niverapine..

OH-Hydroxile group/

OD- Once a day.

PEP-Postexposure prophylaxis.

P450- Cytochromes P450 (CYPs) are proteins of the superfamily of enzimes that use to take part in the hepatic metabolism of the drugs.

RNA- Ribonucleic acid. Is a polymeric molecule essential in various biological processes which are in relation with the process of coding, decoding, regulation, and expression of genes.

RDP-Related Drugs Problems.

RIT- Ritonavir.

SULT1A1- Sulfotransferase 1A1 is an enzyme that in humans is encoded by the *SULT1A1* gene.

TDS-Three times daily.

TDF- Tenofovir

3TC-Lamivudine.

Iu-International units

Ug-Microgram.

Mg-Miligram.

ml-Mililiter.

L-Liter.

Umol/L- Micromol per liter

%- Per cent.

DESCRIPTIONS OF SOME ADVERSE DRUGS REACTIONS OF THE ANTIRETROVIRAL DRUGS

I)-LIPODISTROPHY

The lipodystrophy syndromes is a disease cause by a group of genetic or acquired disorders, in this disease the human body is not able to produce and maintain healthy the fat tissue.

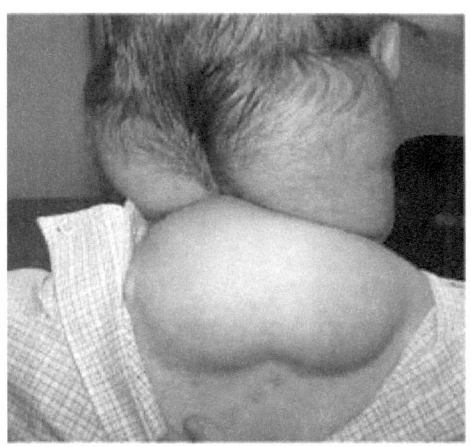

Picture # 1. It shows a patient with lipodystrophy.

Source: data:image/jpeg;base64

II)-GYNECOMASTIA

The Gynecomastia is a disease of the endocrine system; it is a noncancerous disorder that increase the size of the male breast tissue.

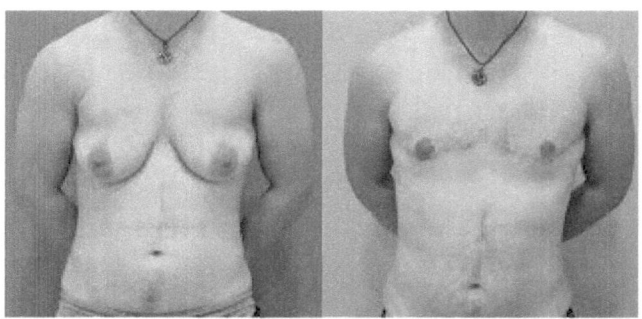

Picture # 2. It shows a patient with gynecomastia.

Source:

https://www.google.com.na/imgres?imgurl=https%3A%2F%2Fwww.wakeplasticsurgery.com

III)-NEPHROTOXICITY

The Nephrotoxicity is a disease related with the toxicity in the kidneys.

IV)-PSYCHOSIS

The psychosis is an abnormal condition of the mind that results in depression, fear, aggressively and another symptoms.

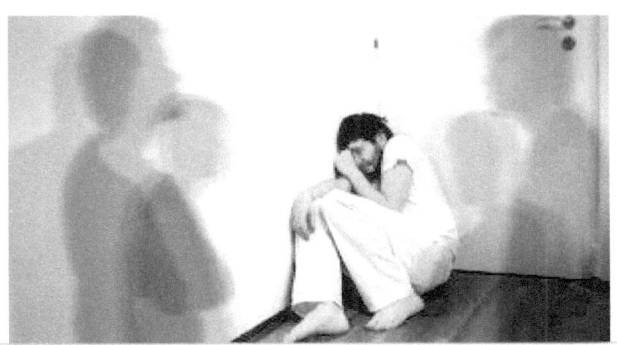

Picture # 3. It shows a patient with gynecomastia.

Source: data:image/jpeg;base64

A GRAFIC TESTIMONY ABOUT HIV AND ITS CONSEQUENCES

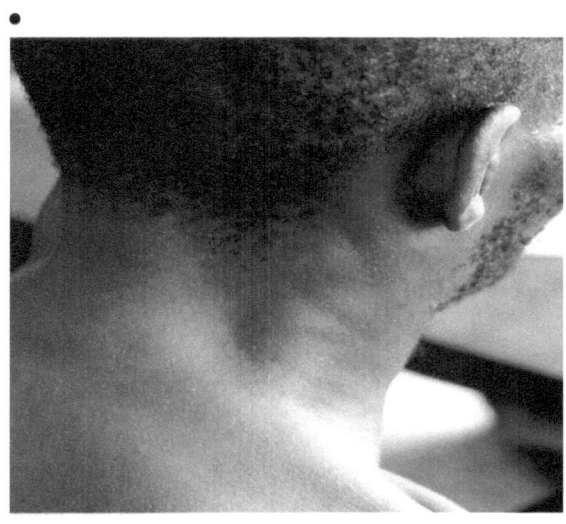

Picture # 1. Persistent generalized lymphadenopathy (PGL)

Source: Courtesy of Charles Steinberg MD

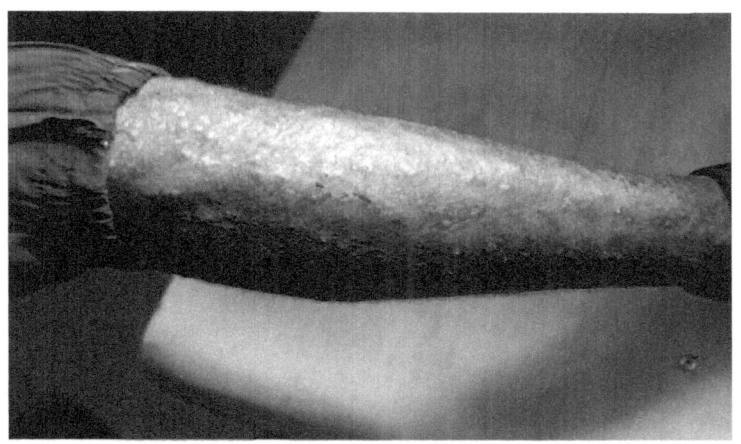

Picture # 2. Pruritic Papular Eruption

Source: Courtesy of Charles Steinberg MD

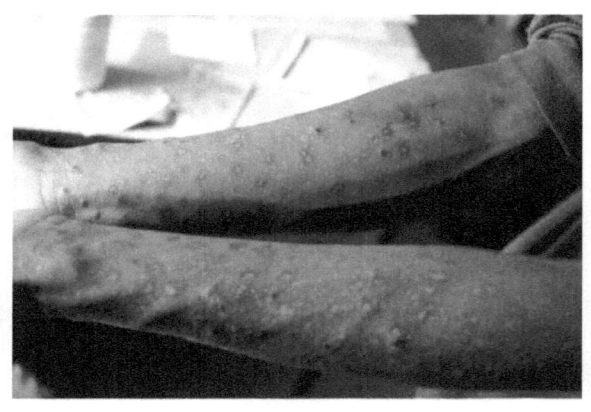

Picture # 3. Pruritic Papular Eruption
Source: Courtesy of Charles Steinberg MD

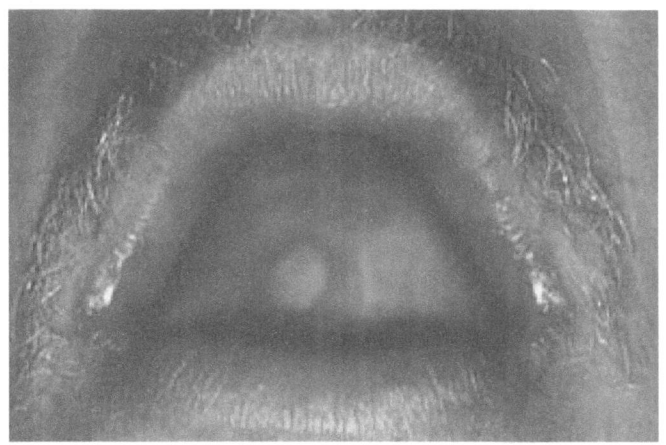

Picture # 4. Apthous Ulcer
Source: www.HIVdent.org. Copyright © 1996-2000 David Reznik, D.D.S

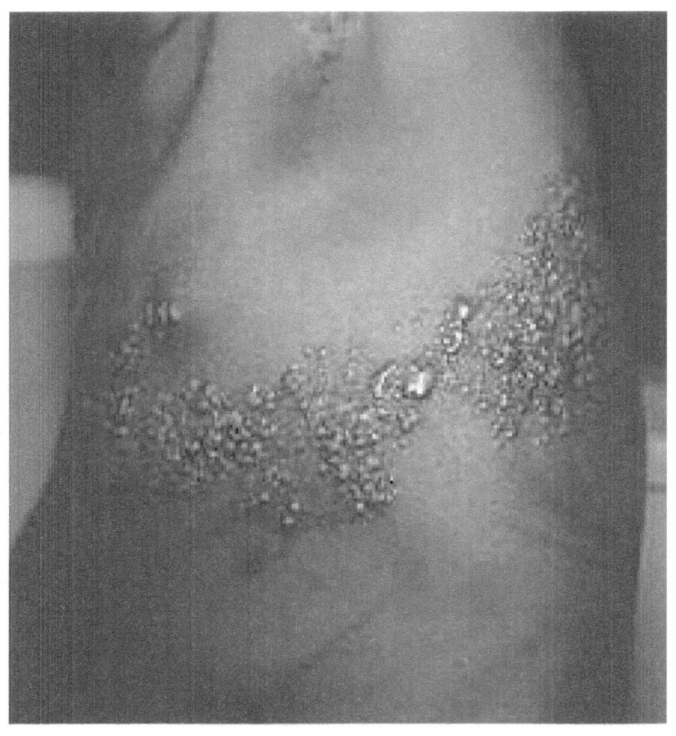

Picture # 5. Herpes Zoster
Source: Courtesy of the Public Health Image Library/CDC

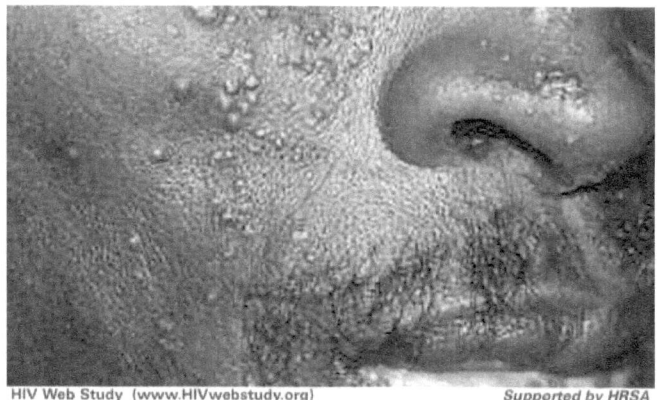

Picture # 6. Molluscum Contagiosum
Source: Courtesy of the Public Health Image Library/CDC

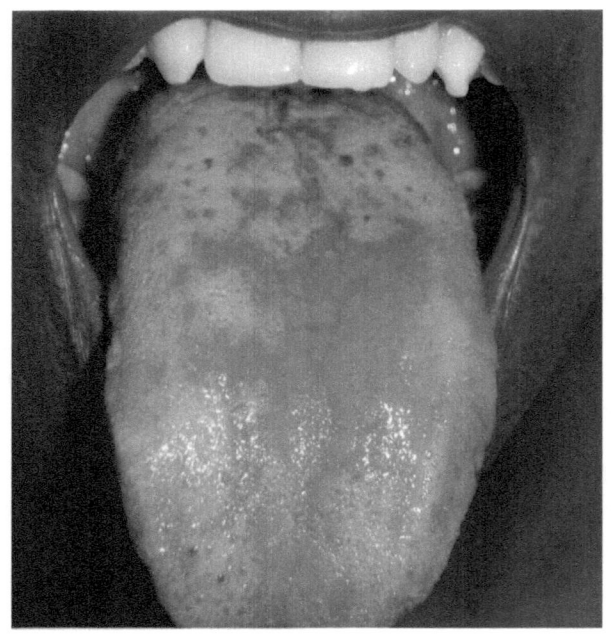

Picture # 7. Oral Candidiasis
Source: Courtesy of Samuel Anderson, MD

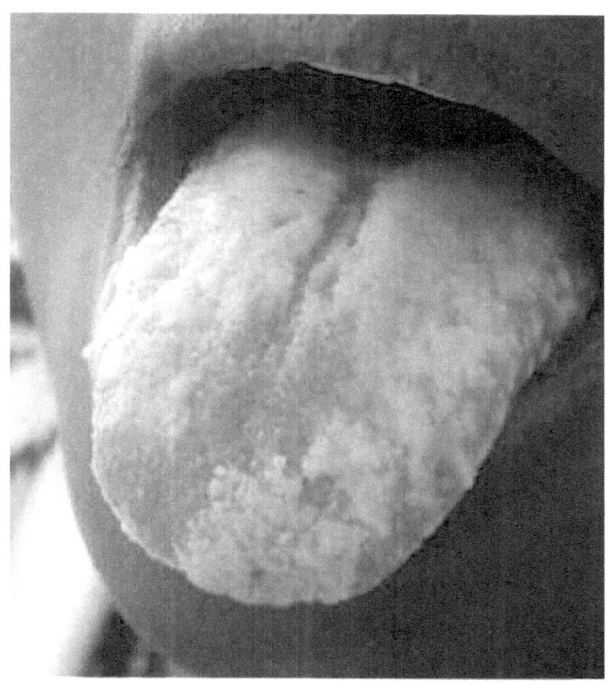

Picture # 8. Oral Candidiasis
Source: Courtesy of Dr. R. Ojoh

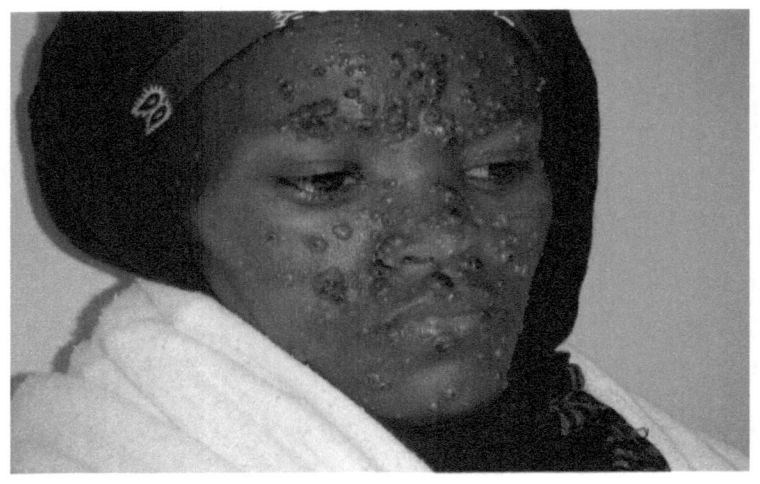

Picture # 9. Disseminated Cutaneous Cryptococcosis
Source: Courtesy of Samuel Anderson, MD

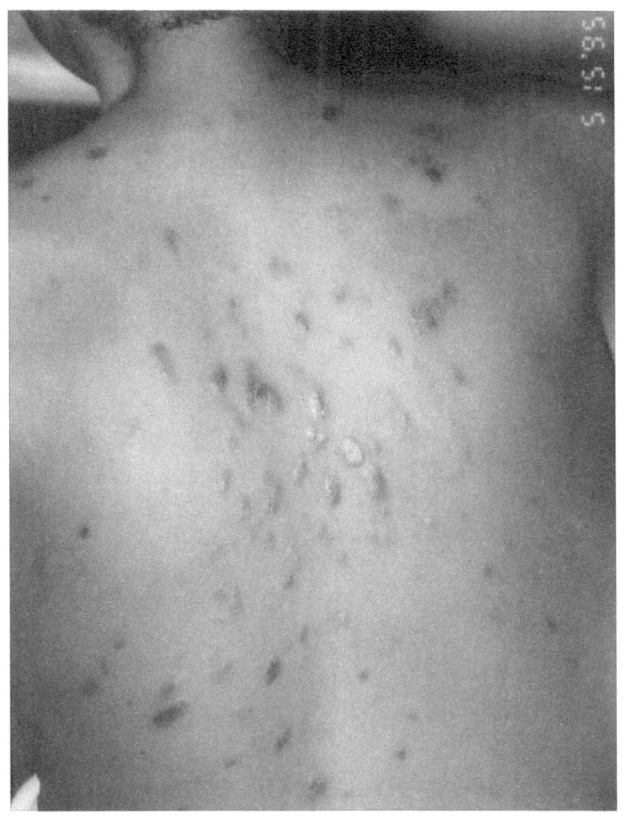

Picture # 10. Kaposi's Sarcoma
Source: Courtesy of Tom Thacher, MD

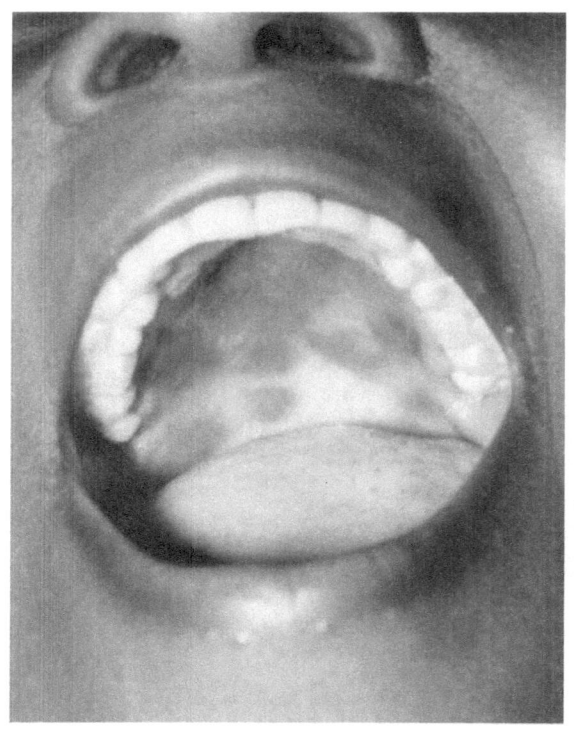

Picture # 11. Kaposi's Sarcoma
Source: Courtesy of Tom Thacher, MD

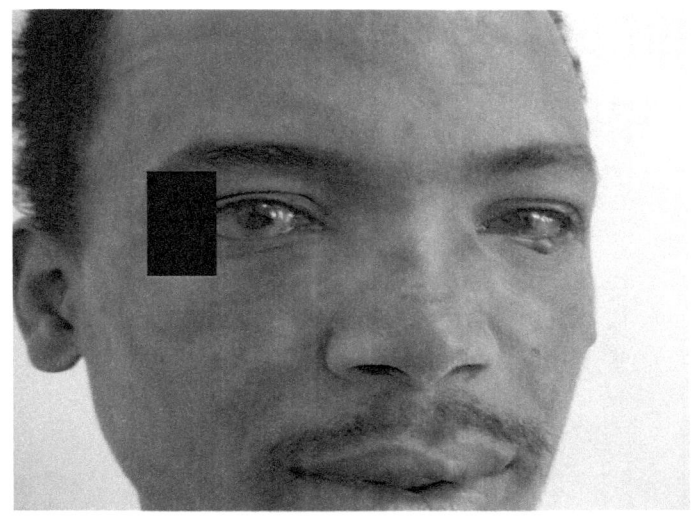

Picture # 12. Kaposi's Sarcoma
Source: Courtesy of Samuel Anderson, MD

About the author

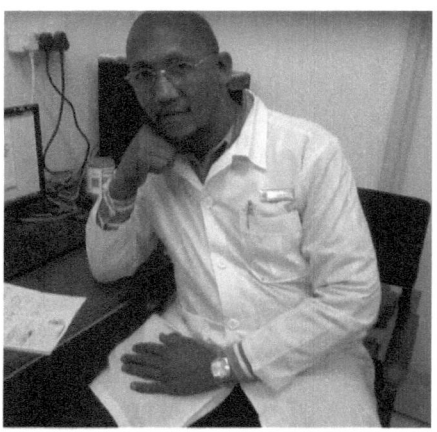

Picture # 1. The author of this book in the pharmacy in the CDC Rundu State Hospital in Kavango east region. Namibia. 2017.

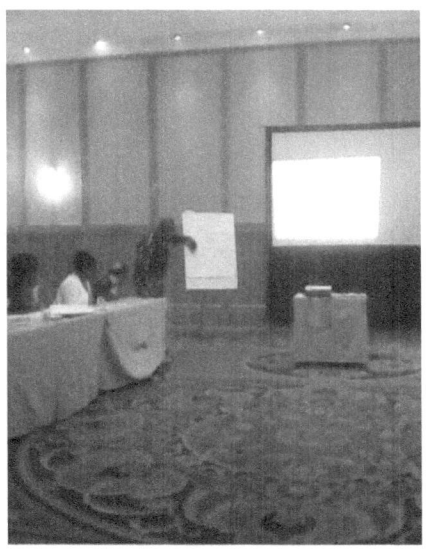

Picture # 2. The author of this book making a presentation in a workshop concerning to the management of the HIV/AIDS. 2016. Namibia.

REFERENCES

1-Munger MA (Nov 2010). "Polypharmacy and combination therapy in the management of hypertens". Drugs Aging. 27: 871–83.doi:10.2165/11538650-000000000-00000 PMID 20964461.

2-"Polypharmacy in Elderly Patients" (PDF). Vumc.nl. Retrieved 16 January 2015.

3. Stawicki, S. P.; Gerlach, A. T. (2009). "Polypharmacy and medication errors: Stop, listen, look, and analyze...". OPUS 12 Scientist. 3 (1): 6–10.

5-Haider, SI; Johnell, K; Thorslund, M; Fastbom, J (2007). "Trends in polypharmacy and potential drug-drug interactions across educational groups in elderly patients in Sweden for the period 1992 - 2002". International Journal of Clinical Pharmacology and Therapeutics.45 (12): 643–653.doi:10.5414/cpp45643. PMID 18184532.

6- Haider, SI; Ansari, Z; Vaughan, L; Matters, H; Emerson, E. (2014). "Prevalence and factors associated with polypharmacy in Victorian adults with intellectual disability". Research in Developmental Disabilities.35

(11): 3070–3080.doi:10.1016/j.ridd.2014.07.060.

7- Da Cruz, Ligiane Paula; Miranda, Patrícia Monforte Miranda; Vedana, Kelly Graziani; Miasso, Adriana Inocenti (2011)."Medication therapy: Adherence, knowledge and difficulties of elderly people from bipolar disorder" (PDF).Revista Latino-Americana De Enfermagem (RLAE).19 (4): 944–952.doi:10.1590/S0104-11692011000400013. PMID 21876947.

8-Gellad, Walid F.; Grenard, Jerry L.; Marcum, Zachary A. (2011)."A systematic review of barriers to medication adherence in the elderly: Looking beyond cost and regimen complexity".American Journal of Geriatric Pharmacotherapy.9 (1): 11–23. doi:10.1016/j.amjopharm.2011.02.004.PMC 3084587.PMID 21459305.

9-Cline, C.M.J.; Björck-Linné, A.K.; Israelsson, B.Y.A.; Willenheimer, R.B.; Erhardt, L.R. (1999-06-01). "Non-compliance and knowledge of prescribed medication in elderly patients with heart failure". European Journal of Heart Failure. 1 (2): 145–149. doi:10.1016/S1388-9842(99)00014-8. ISSN 1879-0844.

10-Yasein, Nada A.; Barghouti, Farihan F.; Irshaid, Yacoub M.; Suleiman, Ahmad A. (March 2013). "Discrepancies between elderly patient's self-reported and prescribed medications: a social investigation".Scandinavian Journal of Caring Sciences.27 (1): 131–138. doi:10.1111/j.1471-6712.2012.01012.x.PMID 22616831.

11-Haider, SI; Johnell, K; Weitoft, GR; Thorslund, M; Fastbom, J (2009). "The influence of educational level on polypharmacy and inappropriate drug use: a register-based study of more than 600,000 older people.".Journal of the American Geriatrics Society.57 (1): 62–69. doi:10.1111/j.1532-5415.2008.02040.x.PMID 19054196.

12-"When Is Polypharmacy an Advantage?". Ajp.psychiatryonline.org. Retrieved 6 January 2015.

13-Sergi, G; De Rui, M; Sarti, S; Manzato, E (2011). "Polypharmacy in the elderly: Can comprehensive geriatric assessment reduce inappropriate medication use?".Drugs Aging.28 (7): 509–518. doi:10.2165/11592010-000000000-00000.

14-Mandell, A.J.; Selz, K.A. (1992). "Dynamical systems in psychiatry: Now what?".Biological Psychiatry.32: 299–301.doi:10.1016/0006-3223(92)90034-w.

15-Callahan, J.; Sashin, J. I. (1987). "Models of affect-response and anorexia nervosa".Ann. N.Y. Acad. Sci. 504: 241–259. doi:10.1111/j.1749-6632.1987.tb48736.x.

15- Qato, DM; Wilder, J; Schumm, LP; Gillet, V; Alexander, GC (2016). "Changes in Prescription and Over-the-Counter Medication and Dietary Supplement Use Among Older Adults in the United States, 2005 vs 2011".JAMA.176 (4): 473–482.doi:10.1001/jamainternmed.2015.8581.

16-Boyd, CM; Darer, J; Boult, C; Fried, LP; Boult, L; Wu, AW (2005). "Clinical practice guidelines and quality of care for older patients with multiple comorbid diseases: implications for pay for performance".JAMA.294 (6): 716–24. doi:10.1001/jama.294.6.716.PMID16091574.

17-Jump up^ Haider, SI; Johnell, K; Thorslund, M; Fastbom, J (2007). "Analysis of the association between polypharmacy and socioeconomic position among elderly aged >/=77 years in Sweden".Clin Ther.32 (2):

419–27. doi:10.1016/j.clinthera.2008.02.010.PMID 18343279.

18-Page, AT; Clifford R., M; Potter, K; Schwartz, D; Etherton-Beer, CD (14 April 2016). "The feasibility and the effect of deprescribing in older adults on mortality and health: A systematic review".British Journal of Clinical Pharmacology.doi:10.1111/bcp.12975.PMID27077231.

19-Potter, Kathleen; Flicker, Leon; Page, Amy; Etherton-Beer, Christopher (4 March 2016)."Deprescribing in frail older people: a randomised controlled trial.".PLoS One.11 (3): e0149984.doi:10.1371/journal.pone.0149984.PMC 4778763 .PMID 26942907.

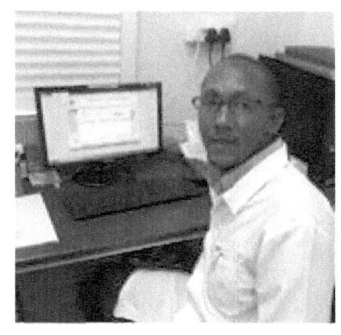

JUAN E. CALDERIN CAMPBELL. Graduated by the Superior Institute of Medical Science of Santiago de Cuba in Cuba as Bachelor degree in pharmaceutical Services. 2012. Graduated as Industrial pharmacist in Cuba in 1994 in the Center for the Engineering Genetic and the Biotechnology with thesis for the process of purification of the recombinants proteins for the elaboration of the HIV test. Graduated by the Superior Institute of Medical Science of Santiago de Cuba with diploma in Pharmacoepidemiology 2014. Author of the book. Medicinal plants and their curatives proprieties. Editorial Oriente Cuba 2013. Author of the book The parasitary and the sexual transmission disease. Editorial científico-tecnica Cuba 2015. Actually pharmacist of the CDC of the Rundu district in the Kavango east región. Namibia.

www.ingramcontent.com/pod-product-compliance
Lightning Source LLC
Chambersburg PA
CBHW020438220526
45464CB00002B/762